I0145971

The Anti-Inflammatory Cookbook for Breakfast

Wake up in the Morning and Fight Body Inflammation With Simple and Delicious Recipes

By
Olga Jones

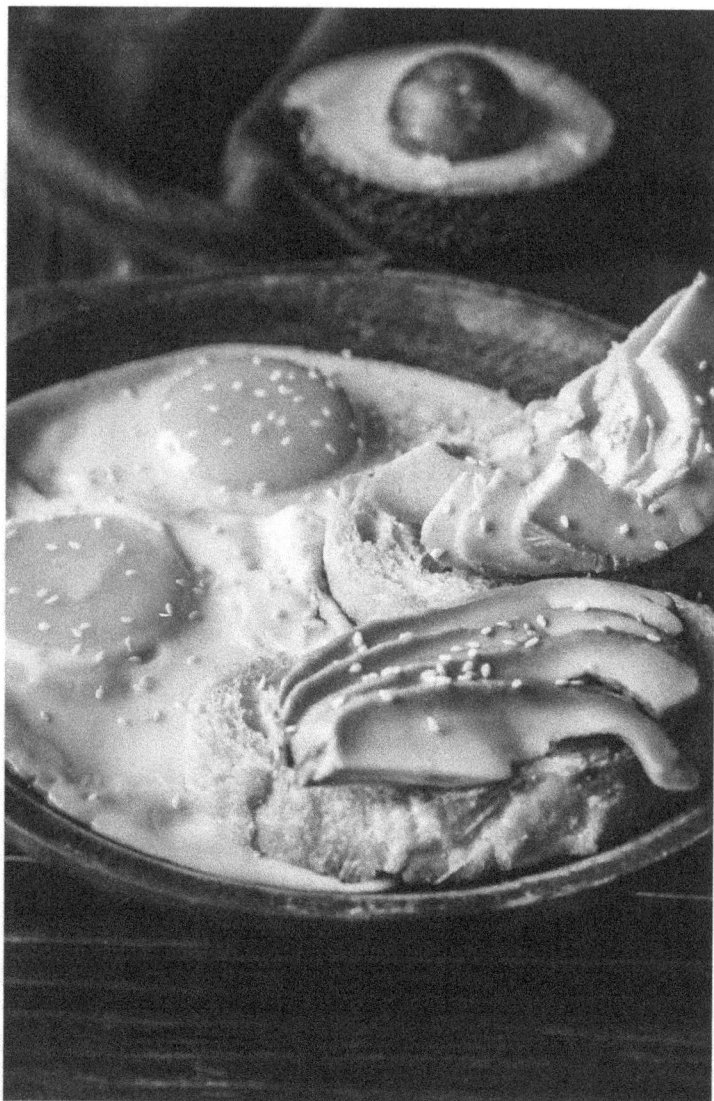

© Copyright 2021 by Olga Jones - All rights reserved.The following Book is reproduced below with the goal of providing information that is as accurate and reliable as possible. Regardless, purchasing this Book can be seen as consent to the fact that both the publisher and the author of this book are in no way experts on the topics discussed within and that any recommendations or suggestions that are made herein are for entertainment purposes only. Professionals should be consulted as needed prior to undertaking any of the action endorsed herein.

This declaration is deemed fair and valid by both the American Bar Association and the Committee of Publishers Association and is legally binding throughout the United States.

Furthermore, the transmission, duplication, or reproduction of any of the following work including specific information will be considered an illegal act irrespective of if it is done electronically or in print. This extends to creating a secondary or tertiary copy of the work or a recorded copy and is only allowed with the express written consent from the Publisher. All additional rights reserved.

The information in the following pages is broadly considered a truthful and accurate account of facts and as such, any inattention, use, or misuse of the information in question by the reader will render any resulting actions solely under their purview. There are no scenarios in which the publisher or the original author of this work can be in any fashion deemed liable for any hardship or damages that may befall them after undertaking information described herein.

Additionally, the information in the following pages is intended only for informational purposes and should thus be thought of as universal. As befitting its nature, it is presented without assurance regarding its prolonged validity or interim quality. Trademarks that are mentioned are done without written consent and can in no way be considered an endorsement from the trademark holder.

Table of Contents

INTRODUCTION

What is the Anti-Inflammatory Diet?

The anti-inflammatory diet is the best choice for your health if you have conditions that cause inflammation. Such conditions are asthma, chronic peptic ulcer, tuberculosis, rheumatoid arthritis, periodontitis, Crohn's disease, sinusitis, active hepatitis, etc. Along with medical treatment, proper nutrition is very important. An anti-inflammatory diet can help to reduce the pain from inflammation for a few notches. Such a diet isn't a panacea but a significant help in any treatment. Inflammation is a natural response of your body to infections, injuries, and illnesses. The classic symptoms of inflammation are redness, pain, heat, and swelling. Nevertheless, some diseases don't have any symptoms. Such illnesses are diabetes, heart disease, cancer, etc. That's why we should care about our health permanently and an anti-inflammatory diet is one of the ways for it.

Inflammation is your immune system's response to injury or unwanted microbes in your body. It is a natural process and vital part of your body's healing process. When inflammation becomes systemic and chronic, however, it becomes a problem, and measures need to be taken. This type of inflammation serves no purpose, and can cause a lot of harm to the body.

This book has a LOT of recipes, and not every recipe might work for you. For example, if you're allergic to dairy or gluten, the recipes containing those ingredients will cause more harm than good. However, substitutions are possible for all of these, so you will be fine following this book as long as you keep an eye on the ingredients and use a bit of creativity where you have to! Once you understand the fundamentals of the diet, you will be fully equipped to create your own recipes from scratch!This is the most important information that you should know before starting a diet. Any diet is not a magic remedy for all diseases; it is a support for the body during a difficult time of treatment. Start your new healthy life from one small step and you will see the huge results within half a year. You can be sure that your body will be thankful to you by giving you a fresh look and energy for new achievements.

Spiced Apple Omelet

Yield: 1 serving

Preparation Time: 10 min

Cooking Time: 10 min

Ingredients:

- 2 large organic eggs
- 1/8 teaspoon organic vanilla flavor
- Pinch of salt
- 2 teaspoons coconut oil, divided
- ½ of the large apple, cored and sliced thinly
- ¼ teaspoon ground cinnamon
- 1/8 teaspoon ground ginger
- 1/8 teaspoon ground nutmeg

Directions:

1. In a bowl, add eggs, vanilla flavoring and salt and beat till fluffy. Keep aside.

2. In a nonstick frying pan, melt 1 teaspoon of coconut oil on medium-low heat.

3. Sprinkle the apple slices with spices evenly made in the pan inside a single layer.

4. Cook for around 4-5 minutes, flipping once inside the middle way.

5. Add the rest of the oil in the skillet.

6. Add the egg mixture over apple slices evenly.

7. Tilt the pan to spread the egg mixture evenly.

8. Cook for approximately 3-4 minutes.

9. Transfer the omelet to a plate and serve.

Baked Oatmeal

Yield: 6 servings

Preparation Time: 15 minutes

Cooking Time: 32-37 minutes

Ingredients:

- 2¼ cups gluten-free rolled oats
- 1½ teaspoons baking powder
- 1½ teaspoons ground cinnamon
- Salt, to taste
- 1/3 cup maple syrup
- 2½ cups unsweetened almond milk
- 2 teaspoons organic vanilla flavoring
- 2½ cups carrots, peeled and shredded
- 1½ teaspoons fresh ginger, grated finely
- ½ cup walnuts, chopped
- ¼ cup raisins

Directions:

1. Preheat the oven to 375 degrees F. Grease a 11x8-inch casserole dish.

2. In a large bowl, mix together oats, baking powder, cinnamon and salt.

3. In another bowl, add maple syrup, almond milk and vanilla extract.

4. Add oats mixture into almond milk mixture and mix till well combined.

5. Fold in carrots and ginger.

6. Transfer a combination into prepared casserole dish.

7. Top with raisins and walnuts evenly.

8. Bake for approximately 32-37 minutes.

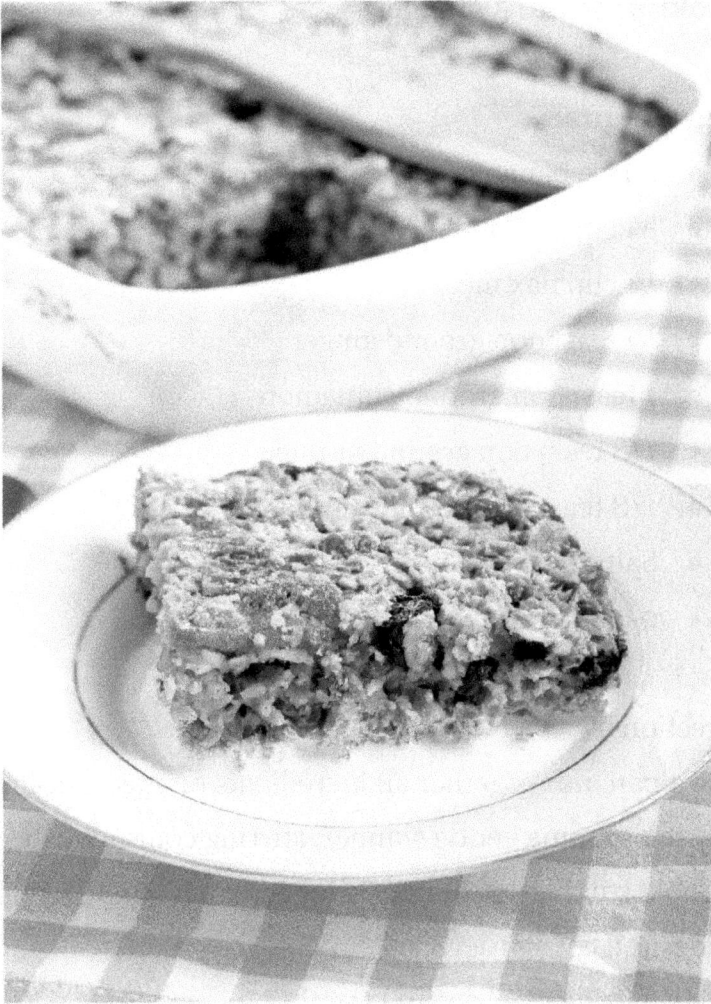

Banana Porridge

Yield: 2-4 servings

Preparation Time: 10 minutes

Cooking Time: 5 minutes

Ingredients:

- 2 ripe bananas, peeled and mashed
- ¾ cup almond meal
- ¼ cup flax meal
- ½ teaspoon ground ginger
- 1 teaspoon ground cinnamon
- 1/8 teaspoon ground nutmeg
- 1/8 teaspoon ground cloves
- Salt, to taste
- 2 cups coconut milk

Directions:

1. In a pan, mix together all ingredients on medium-low heat.

2. Bring to some gentle simmer, stirring continuously.

3. Cook, stirring continuously for approximately 2-3 minutes or till desired consis10cy.

4. Serve using your desired topping.

Ham & Bell Pepper Muffins

Yield: 4 servings

Preparation Time: 10 minutes

Cooking Time: 18-twenty or so minutes

Ingredients:
- 8 organic eggs
- Salt and freshly ground black pepper, to taste
- 2 tablespoons water
- 8-ounces cooked ham, crumbled
- 1 cup red bell pepper, seeded and chopped
- 1 cup onion, chopped

Directions:
1. Preheat the oven to 350 degrees F. Grease 8 cups of your muffin tray.

2. In a bowl, add eggs, salt, black pepper and water and beat till well combined.

3. Stir in ham, bell pepper and onion.

4. Transfer a combination in prepared muffin cups evenly.

5. Bake for about 18-20 min or till a toothpick inserted inside the center comes out clean.

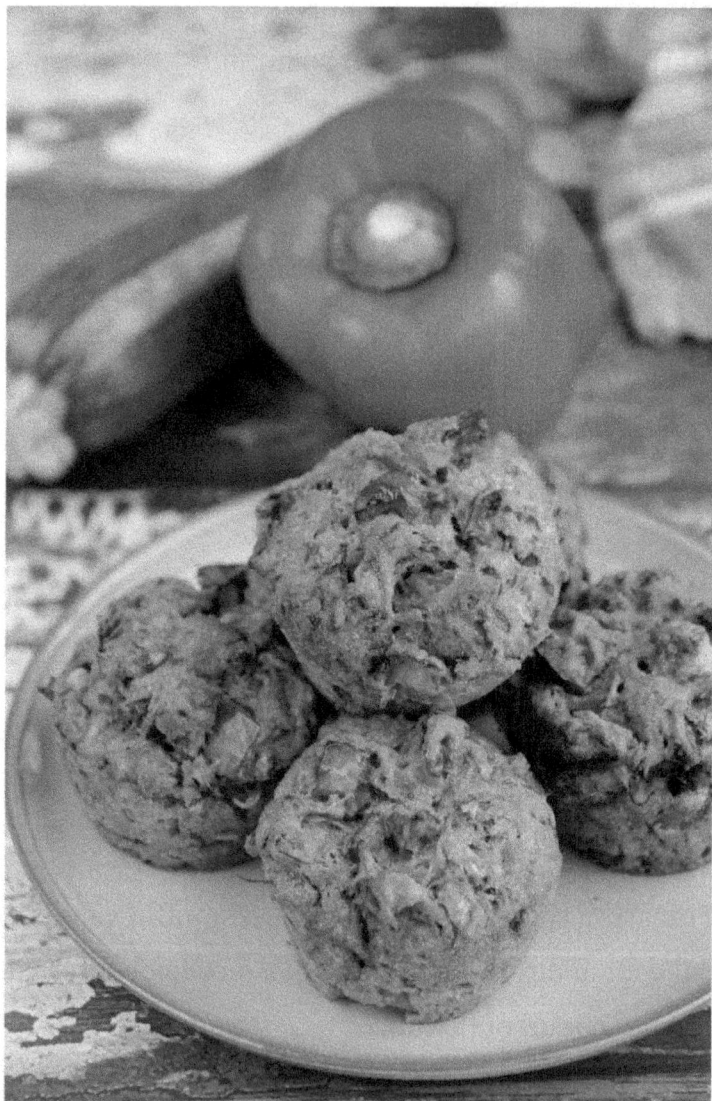

Eggs In Avocado Cup

Yield: 2 servings

Preparation Time: 10 minutes

Cooking Time: 15-20 min

Ingredients:
- 2 ripe avocados, halved, pitted and scooped out about 2 tablespoons of flesh
- 4 organic eggs
- Salt and freshly ground black pepper, to taste
- 1 tablespoon chives, minced

Directions:
1. Preheat the oven to 425 degrees F.

2. Arrange the avocado halves in a small baking dish.

3. In a smaller bowl, break an egg after which carefully transfer it within an avocado half.

4. Repeat with remaining eggs.

5. Bake approximately 15-twenty minutes or till desired doneness.

6. Serve immediately with all the sprinkling of salt, black pepper and chives.

Veggie Poached Eggs

Yield: 4 servings

Preparation Time: 10 min

Cooking Time: quarter-hour

Ingredients:

- 2 tablespoons olive oil, divided
- 1 pound zucchini, quartered and sliced thinly
- 1 large red bell pepper, seeded and chopped
- 1 medium onion, chopped
- 1 teaspoon fresh rosemary, chopped finely
- Salt, to taste
- 4 large organic eggs
- Freshly ground black pepper, to taste

Directions:

1. In a big skillet, heat 1 tablespoon of oil on medium-high heat.

2. Add zucchini, bell pepper and onion and sauté for approximately 5-8 minutes.

3. Stir in rosemary and salt. With a wooden spoon, create a large well inside the center of skillet by moving the veggie mixture on the sides.

4. Reduce the warmth to medium. Pour remaining oil inside well.

5. Carefully, crack the eggs within the well. Sprinkle the eggs with salt and black pepper.

6. Cook for approximately 1- 2 minutes. Cover the skillet and cook approximately 1-2 minutes more.

7. For serving, carefully, scoop the veggie mixture in 4 serving plates. Top with an egg and serve.

Apple Omelet

Yield: 1 serving

Preparation Time: 10 min

Cooking Time: 9 minutes

Ingredients:
- 2 teaspoons coconut oil, divided
- ½ of enormous green apple, cored and sliced thinly
- ¼ teaspoon ground cinnamon
- 1/8 teaspoon ground nutmeg
- 2 large organic eggs
- 1/8 teaspoon organic vanilla extract
- Pinch of salt
- Maple syrup, if desired

Directions:

1. In a nonstick frying pan, heat 1 teaspoon of oil on medium-low heat.

2 Add apple slices and sprinkle with nutmeg and cinnamon.

3. Cook for approximately 4-5 minutes, turning once inside middle.

4. Meanwhile inside a bowl, add eggs, vanilla and salt and beat till fluffy.

5. Add remaining oil inside the pan and let it melt completely.

6. Place the egg mixture over apple slices evenly.

7. Cook for approximately 3-4 minutes or till desired doneness.

8. Carefully, turn the pan over a serving plate and immediately, fold the omelet.

9. Serve while using drizzling of maple syrup if you like.

No-Bake Veggie Frittata

Yield: 4 servings

Preparation Time: 10 minutes

Cooking Time: 26 minutes

Ingredients:
- 2 tablespoons coconut oil
- 1 large sweet potato, peeled and cut into thin slices
- 1 red bell pepper, seeded and sliced
- 2 zucchinis, sliced
- 8 organic eggs
- Salt and freshly ground black pepper, to taste
- 2 tablespoons fresh parsley, chopped finely

Directions:
1. Preheat the oven to broiler.

2. In a substantial oven proof skillet, heat oil on medium-low heat.

3. Add sweet potato and cook for approximately 7-8 minutes.

4. Add bell pepper and zucchini and cook for about 3-4 minutes.

5. Meanwhile in a bowl, add eggs, salt and black pepper and beat till well combined.

6. Pour egg mixture over veggies evenly. Immediately, decrease the heat to low.

7. Cook for about 10 minutes or till just done.

8. Transfer the skillet beneath the broiler and broil approximately 3-4 minutes or till top becomes golden brown.

9. Cut the frittata in desired size slices. Serve while using garnishing of parsley.

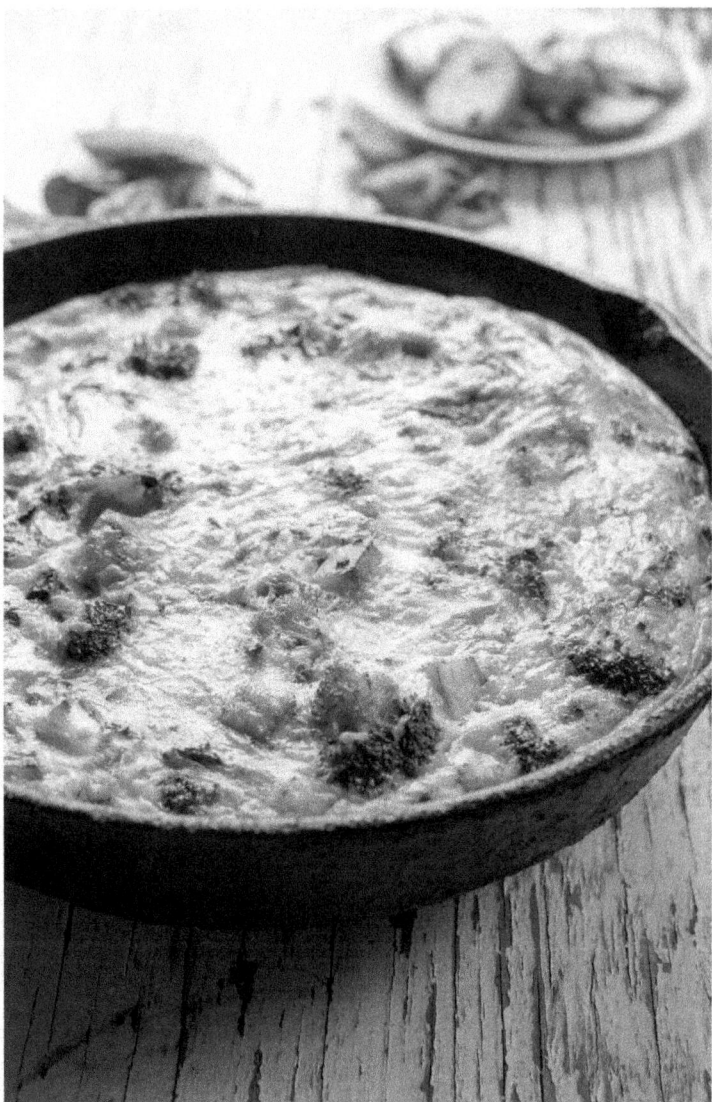

Almond Mascarpone Dumplings

Time To Prepare: ten minutes

Time to Cook: ten minutes

Yield: Servings 6

Ingredients:
- ¼ cup ground almonds
- ¼ cup honey
- 1 cup all-purpose unbleached flour
- 1 cup whole-wheat flour
- 1 tablespoon butter
- 1 teaspoon extra-virgin olive oil
- 2 teaspoons apple juice
- 3 ounces mascarpone cheese
- 4 egg whites

Directions:
1. Strain together both types of flour in a big container.

2. Stir in the almonds.

3. In a different container, whisk together the egg whites, cheese, oil, and juice on moderate speed using an electric mixer.

4. Place the flour, and egg white mixture with a dough hook on moderate speed or using your hands until a dough forms.

5. Boil 1 gallon water in a medium-size saucepot.

6. Take a scoop of dough and use a second spoon to push it into the boiling water.

7. Cook up to the dumpling floats to the top, minimum 5 to ten minutes.

8. You can cook several dumplings at once — just take care not to crowd the pot.

9. Take off using a slotted spoon and drain using paper towels. Warm a medium-size sauté pan on moderate to high heat.

10. Put in the butter, then put the dumplings in the pan and cook until light brown. Set on serving plates and sprinkle with honey.

Almond Scones

Time To Prepare: ten minutes

Time to Cook: twenty minutes

Yield: Servings 6

Ingredients:

- 1 cup almonds
- ¼ cup arrowroot flour
- 1 tablespoon coconut flour
- 1 teaspoon ground turmeric Salt, to taste
- Freshly ground black pepper, to taste
- 1 egg
- ¼ cup essential olive oil
- 3 tablespoons raw honey
- 1 teaspoon vanilla flavoring
- 1 1/3 cups almond flour

Directions:

1. In a mixer, put almonds then pulse till chopped roughly

2. Move the chopped almonds in a big container.

3. Put flour and spices and mix thoroughly.

4. In another container, put the rest of the ingredients and beat till well blended.

5. Place the flour mixture into the egg mixture then mix till well blended.

6. Position a plastic wrap over the cutting board. Put the dough over the cutting board. Use both your hands to pat into a 1-inch thick circle. Chop the circle in 6 wedges.

7. Set the scones onto a cookie sheet in a single layer. Bake for minimum fifteen-20 minutes.

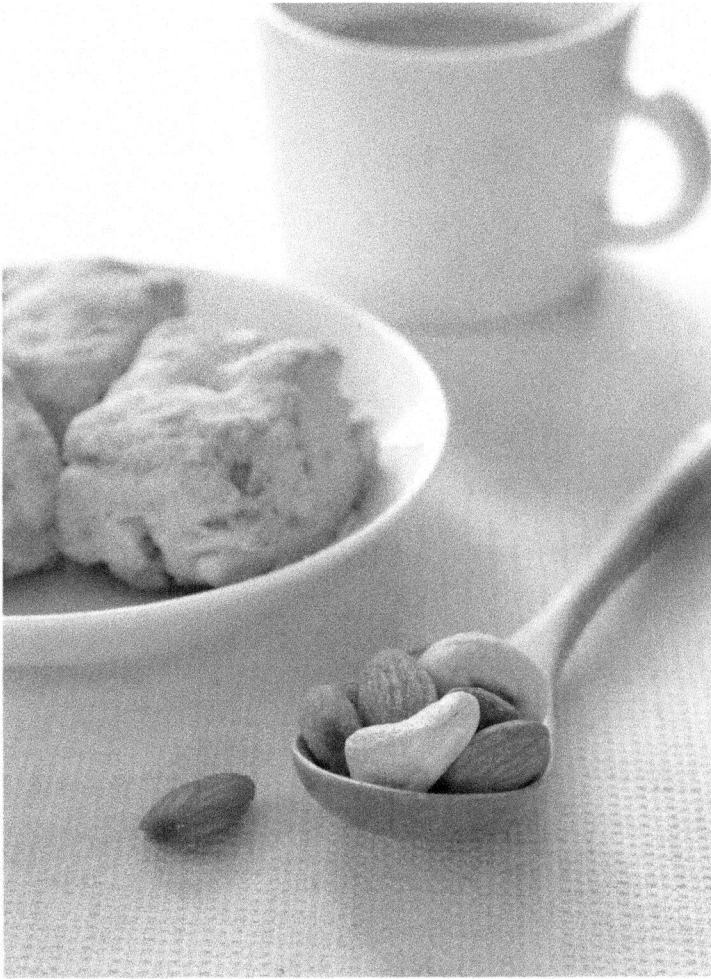

Apple Bread

Time To Prepare: twenty-five minutes

Time to Cook: 1 hour and ten minutes

Yield: Servings 8

Ingredients:

- ¼ tsp. baking powder
- 1 cup peeled, chopped apples
- 1 packet yeast
- 1 tbsp. cinnamon mixed with 1 tablespoon sugar
- 1 tsp. Salt
- 1¾ cups all-purpose flour
- 1¾ cups whole-wheat flour
- 11/3 cups warm water
- 3 tbsp. sugar
- 3 tbsp. tender butter

Directions:

1. Mix yeast, ½ teaspoon sugar, and 1/3 cup water in a container. Allow to sit for five minutes.

2. In a mixing container, put together remaining water, butter, remaining sugar, salt, and baking powder then mix.

3. Mix in the all-purpose flour, then the yeast mixture using an electric mixer. Place the whole-wheat flour.

4. Knead the dough hook for a minimum ten minutes.

5. Place the dough into an oiled container. Cover then rises in a warm place for a minimum of a couple of hours until doubled in bulk.

6. Punch down the dough, then form into a rectangle. Spread the apples on the dough and dust with the cinnamon sugar. Roll into a cylinder and put in an oiled loaf pan.

7. Cover and allow it to rise in a warm oven for 90 minutes until doubled in size.

8. Preheat your oven to 350°F. Uncover the bread and bake for about fifty minutes.

Apple Oatmeal

Time To Prepare: ten minutes

Time to Cook: five minutes

Yield: Servings 2

Ingredients:

- ¼ cup fresh apple juice
- 1 chopped apple, (unpeeled or peeled)
- 1 cup of any non-fat milk, coconut milk or almond milk (not necessary)
- 1 cup water
- 1 teaspoon ground cinnamon
- 2/3 cups rolled oats

Directions:

1. Put the water, juice, and the apple in a deep pot. Bring to boil on moderate heat.

2. Put in the oats and cinnamon. Bring to another boil. Reduce the heat temperature and allow it to simmer for about three minutes or until it is thick.

3. Split the serving into two and serve with milk.

Bake Apple Turnover

Time To Prepare: thirty minutes

Time to Cook: twenty-five minutes

Yield: Servings 4

Ingredients:

- ½ cup palm sugar, crumbled using your hands to loosen granules
- ½ tsp. cinnamon powder
- 1 egg white, whisked in 1 frozen puff pastry, thawed 1 Tbsp. almond flour 2 Tbsp. water
- 4 apples, peeled, cored, diced into bite-sized pieces
- All-purpose flour, for rolling out the dough For the egg wash For the turnovers

Directions:

1. To make the filling: mix almond flour, cinnamon powder, and palm sugar until these resemble coarse meal.

2. Toss in diced apples until thoroughly coated. Set aside

3. On a mildly floured surface, roll the puff pastry until ¼ inch thin. Cut into 8 pieces of 4" x 4" squares. Split prepared apples into 8 equivalent portions. Ladle on individual puff pastry squares. Fold in half diagonally. Push edges to secure.

4. Put each filled pastry on a baking tray coated with parchment paper. Make sure there is ample space between pastries.

5. Freeze for a minimum of twenty minutes, or till ready to bake.

6. Preheat your oven to 400°F or 205°C for ten minutes.

7. Brush frozen pastries with egg wash.

8. Bring in a hot oven, and cook for twelve to fifteen minutes, or until these turn golden brown all over.

9. Take off the baking tray in your oven instantly. Cool slightly for easier handling. Put 1 apple turnover on a plate. Serve warm.

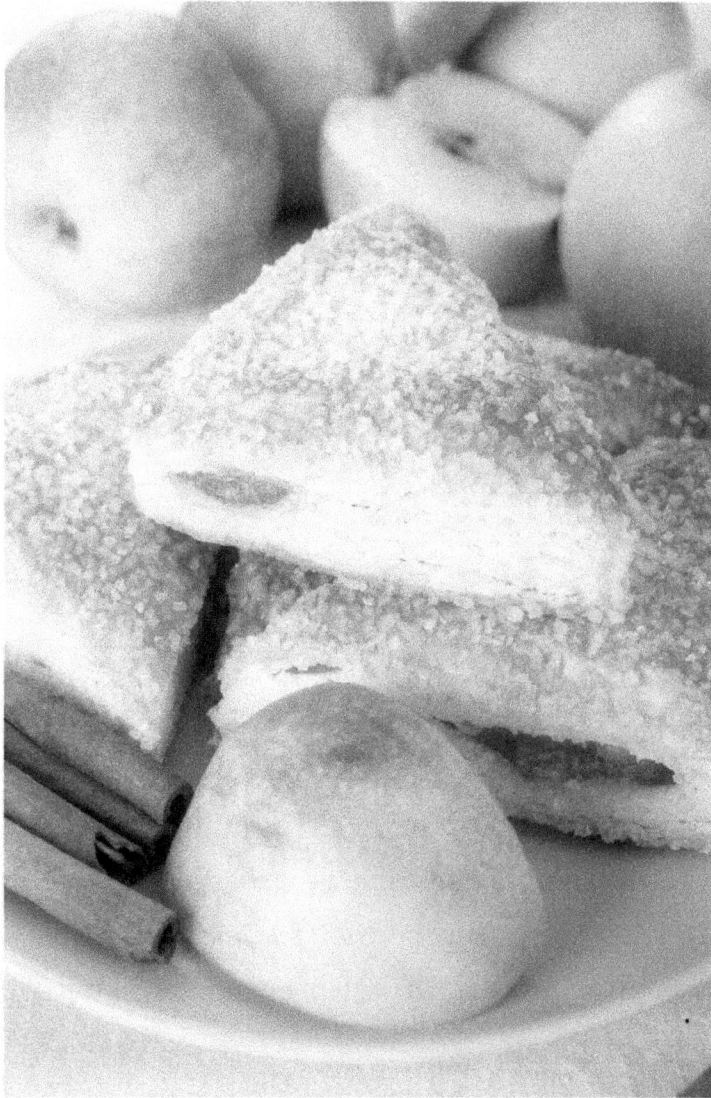

Banana Cashew Toast

Time To Prepare: ten minutes

Time to Cook: 0 minutes

Yield: Servings 3

Ingredients:

- 1 cup roasted cashews (unsalted)
- 2 ripe moderate-sized bananas
- 2 tsp. flax meals
- 2 tsp. honey
- 4 pieces oat bread
- Dash of salt Pinch of cinnamon

Directions:

1. Peel and slice the bananas into ½-inch pieces.

2. Toast the bread.

3. Use a food processor to puree the salt and cashews until they are smooth.

4. Use the puree as a spread on the toasts.

5. On top of the spread, position a layer of bananas.

6. Put in flax meals and a dash of cinnamon on top of the bananas.

7. Top the toast with honey.

Grams Banana-Oatmeal Vegan Pancakes

Time To Prepare: five minutes

Time to Cook: five minutes

Yield: Servings 12

Ingredients:

- ½ c. organic whole wheat flour
- ½ tsp. sea salt
- 1¼ c. old fashioned oats
- 1½ c. soymilk
- 2 ripe bananas
- 2 tsp. Baking powder

Directions:

1. To begin, heat griddle or frying pan on moderate heat.

2. After this, place all ingredients, apart from the banana, into a blender and process until the desired smoothness is achieved.

3. Put in the bananas to blender and blend until the desired smoothness is achieved.

4. Lightly grease griddle with olive or coconut oil, then pour ¼ c. of batter onto griddle and cook for minimum two to three minutes, then flip and cook for approximately 2 minutes or maximum until the pancake is golden brown and thoroughly cooked.

5. Repeat the process with the remaining batter.

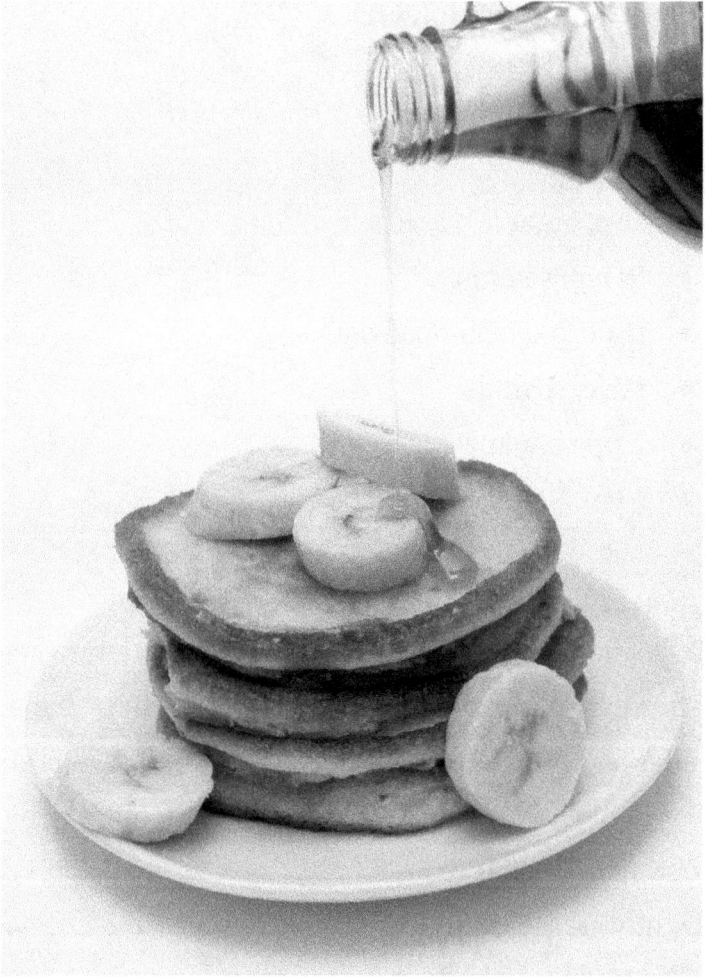

Beef Breakfast Casserole

Time To Prepare: ten minutes

Time to Cook: thirty minutes

Yield: Servings 5

Ingredients:

- ¼ cup cut black olives
- ½ cup Pico de Gallo
- 1 cup baby spinach
- 1 pound of ground beef
- Cooked 10 eggs
- Freshly ground black pepper

Directions:

1. Preheat your oven to 350 degrees Fahrenheit.

2. Prepare a 9" glass pie plate with non-stick spray.

3. Whisk the eggs until frothy.

4. Sprinkle with salt and pepper.

5. Layer the cooked ground beef, Pico de Gallo, and spinach in the pie plate.

6. Slowly pour the eggs over the top.

7. Top with black olives.

8. Bake for minimum 30 minutes, until firm in the center.

9. Cut into 5 pieces before you serve.

Blueberry-Bran Breakfast Sundae

Time To Prepare: ten minutes

Time to Cook: 0 minutes

Yield: Servings 2

Ingredients:

- 1/4 c. fresh blueberries
- 2 c. bran flakes
- 2 c. vanilla or lemon-flavored low-fat yogurt (if possible Greek yogurt) or flavor of choice.
- 2 tbsp. chopped pecans (or nuts of choice)
- 2 tbsp. cut almonds (or nuts of choice)
- 2 tbsp. dried cranberries (or dried or fresh fruit of choice)

Directions:

1. In a container, place 1 c. yogurt, and one c. bran flakes.

2. Top with 1/8 c. fresh blueberries, followed by 1 tbsp.

3. Each of cut almonds, chopped pecans, and dried cranberries.

4. Repeat using the rest of the ingredients to make a second serving. Serve instantly.

Breakfast Pitas

Time To Prepare: 4 minutes

Time to Cook: six minutes

Yield: Servings 4

Ingredients:
- 1 c. raw spinach (cook if you prefer)
- 1 tsp. garlic powder
- 1 tsp. onion powder
- 2 c. bell peppers, chopped (any color)
- 2 tsp. extra virgin olive oil
- 4 whole-wheat pita pockets
- 8 egg whites

Directions:
1. Place the olive oil to a big sauté pan and place on moderate heat.

2. When the oil is hot and shiny, throw in the bell pepper and sauté for approximately 3 minutes or until soft.

3. Put in the spinach now (if you wish it cooked) and sauté for approximately 1 to three minutes or just until the sides begin to wilt.

4. Put the egg whites into a small container, whisk well.

5. Put in spices; whisk well.

6. Pour the egg mixture into the sauté pan and scramble everything together.

7. Turn off the heat and stuff ½ to 1 c. mixture into a pita pocket before you serve.

Carrot Bread

Time To Prepare: ten minutes

Time to Cook: 1 hour

Yield: Servings 8

Ingredients:
- ¼ cup sultanas
- ½-inch piece of fresh ginger, peeled and grated
- 1 tablespoon apple cider vinegar
- 1 tablespoon cumin seeds
- 1 teaspoon organic baking powder
- 2 cups almond meal
- 2 tablespoons macadamia nut oil
- 3 cups carrot, peeled and grated
- 3 organic eggs
- Salt, to taste

Directions:
1. Set the oven to 35 F, then line a loaf pan using parchment paper.

2. In a big container, put together the almond meal, baking powder, cumin seeds, and salt and mix.

3. In another container, put in eggs, nut oil, and vinegar and beat till well blended.

4. Place the egg mixture into the flour mixture and mix till well blended.

5. Fold in the rest of the ingredients.

6. Put the mixture into the prepared loaf pan equally. Bake for approximately 1 hour

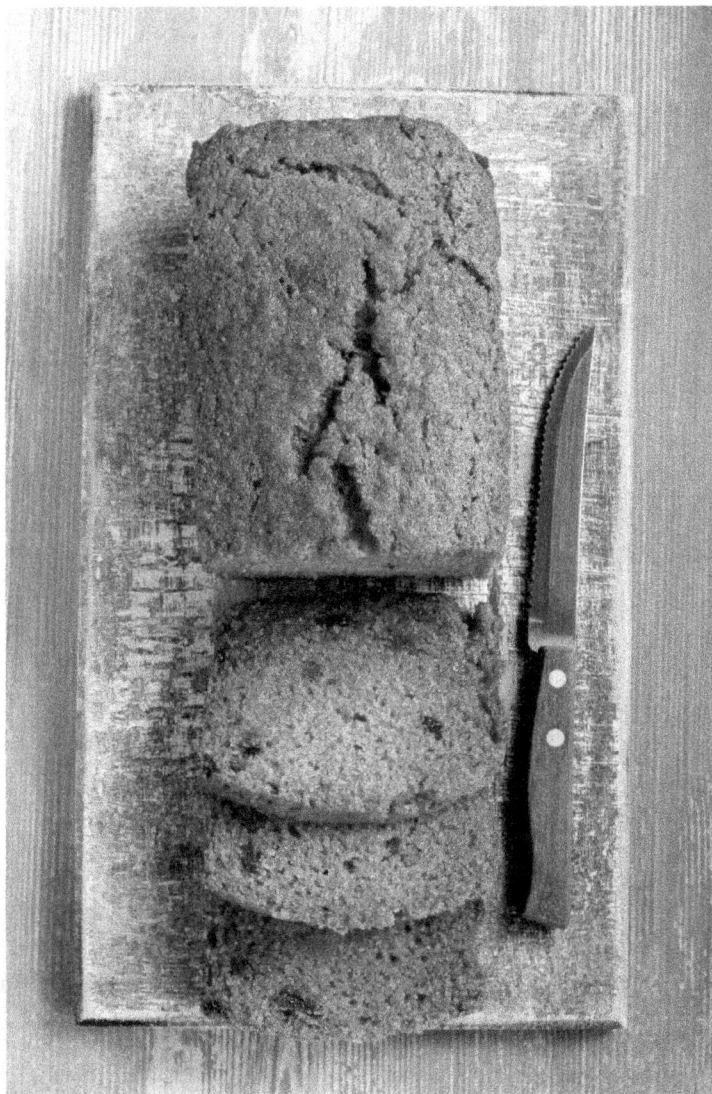

Cauliflower and Chorizo

Time To Prepare: 55 minutes

Time to Cook: forty minutes

Yield: Servings 4

Ingredients:

- ½ teaspoon garlic powder
- 1 cauliflower head; florets separated
- 1 pound chorizo; chopped.
- 1 yellow onion; chopped.
- 12 ounces canned green chilies; chopped.
- 2 tablespoons green onions; chopped.
- 4 eggs; whisked
- Salt and black pepper to the taste.

Directions:

1. Heat a pan on moderate heat; put the chorizo and onion; stir and brown for a few minutes

2. Put in green chilies, stir, cook for a few minutes and take off the heat.

3. In your food processor, mix cauliflower with some salt and pepper and blend.

4. Move this to a container, put in eggs, salt, pepper, and garlic powder and whisk everything.

5. Put in chorizo mix as well, whisk again and move everything to a greased baking dish.

6. Bake using your oven at 375F then bake for at least forty minutes.

7. Leave casserole to cool down for a few minutes, drizzle green onions on top, slice and serve

Cheesy Flax and Hemp Seeds Muffins

Time To Prepare: five minutes

Time to Cook: thirty minutes

Yield: Servings 2

Ingredients:
- ¼ cup almond meal
- ¼ cup cottage cheese, low-fat
- ¼ cup grated parmesan cheese
- ¼ cup raw hemp seeds
- ¼ cup scallion, cut thinly
- ¼ tsp baking powder
- 1 tbsp. olive oil
- 1/8 cup flax seeds meal
- 1/8 cup nutritional yeast flakes
- 3 organic eggs, beaten
- Salt, to taste

Directions:

1. Switch on the oven, then set it 360°F and allow it to preheat.

2. In the meantime, take two ramekins, grease them with oil, and set aside until required.

3. Take a medium container, put in flax seeds, hemp seeds, and almond meal, and then mix in salt and baking powder until combined.

4. Crack eggs in a different container, put in yeast, cottage cheese, and parmesan, stir thoroughly until blended, and then stir this mixture into the almond meal mixture until blended.

5. Fold in scallions, then spread the mixture between prepared ramekins and bake for thirty minutes until muffins are firm and the top is nicely golden brown.

6. When finished, take out the muffins from the ramekins and allow them to cool to room temperature on a wire rack.

7. For meal prepping, wrap each muffin using a paper towel and place in your fridge for maximum thirty-four days.

8. When ready to eat, reheat muffins in the microwave until hot and then serve.

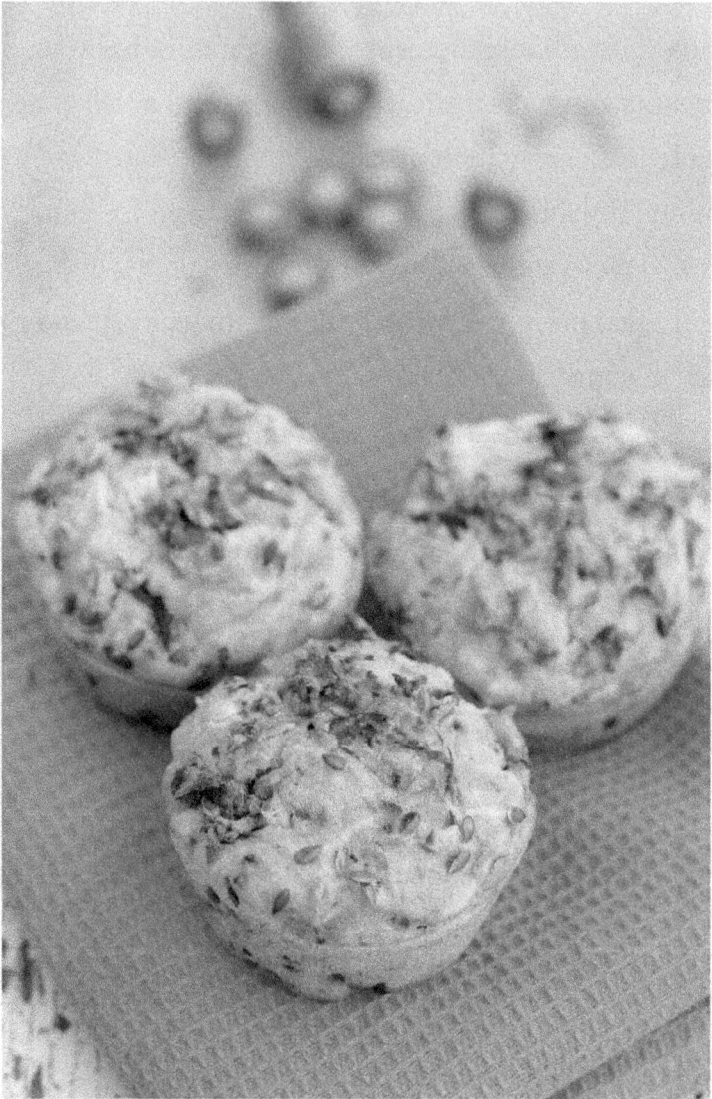

Grams Chicken Muffins

Time To Prepare: 1 hour ten minutes

Time to Cook: thirty minutes

Yield: Servings 3

Ingredients:

- ½ teaspoon garlic powder
- 2 tablespoons green onions; chopped.
- 3 tablespoons hot sauce mixed with 3 tablespoons melted coconut oil
- 3/4 pound chicken breast; boneless
- 6 eggs
- Salt and black pepper to the taste.

Directions:

1. Season chicken breast with pepper, salt, and garlic powder, place on a lined baking sheet, and bake in your oven at 425F for a minimum of twenty-five minutes.

2. Move chicken breast to a container, shred using a fork, and mix with half of the hot sauce and melted coconut oil.

3. Toss to coat and leave aside.

4. In a container, mix eggs with salt, pepper, green onions, and the remaining hot sauce mixed with oil and whisk very well.

5. Split this mix into a muffin tray, top each with shredded chicken, introduce in your oven at 350F then bake for minimum 30 minutes.

6. Serve your muffins hot.

Cilantro Pancakes

Time To Prepare: ten minutes

Time to Cook: 6-8 minutes

Yield: Servings 6

Ingredients:

- ¼ teaspoon ground turmeric
- ½ cup almond flour
- ½ cup fresh cilantro, chopped
- ½ cup tapioca flour
- ½ of red onion, chopped
- ½ teaspoon chili powder
- 1 (½- inch) fresh ginger piece, grated finely
- 1 cup full-Fat coconut milk
- 1 Serrano pepper, minced
- Freshly ground black pepper, to taste Oil, as required Salt, to taste

Directions:

1. In a big container, put together the flours and spices then mix.

2. Place the coconut milk and mix till well blended.

3. Fold within the onion, ginger, Serrano pepper, and cilantro.

4. Lightly, grease a sizable nonstick frying pan with oil and warmth on medium-low heat.

5. Put in about ¼ cup of mixture and tilt the pan to spread it uniformly inside the frying pan.

6. Cook for about four minutes from either side.

7. Repeat with all the rest of the mixture. Serve together with your desired topping.

Cinnamon-Apple Granola with Greek Yogurt

Time To Prepare: five minutes

Time to Cook: ten minutes

Yield: Servings 2

Ingredients:

- ½ apple, peeled and diced
- ½ c. raw almonds, chopped (or raw nuts of choice)
- ½ c. raw walnuts, chopped (or raw nuts of choice)
- 1 cup Greek plain or vanilla yogurt (or flavor of choice)
- 1 tbsp. almond flour
- 1 tsp. ground cinnamon
- 1/16 tsp. vanilla extract
- 1/8 c. applesauce, unsweetened preferred
- 2 tbsp. vanilla
- Protein powder
- 2 tsp. almond butter
- 2 tsp. honey dash of sea salt

Directions:

1. In a mixing container, mix the chopped almonds, chopped walnuts (or preferred raw nuts), diced apple, vanilla Protein powder, almond flour, lucuma (opt), and cinnamon and salt in a container.

2. Mix thoroughly. In a second container, mix the apple sauce, almond butter, honey, and vanilla extract.

3. Mix thoroughly. Pour the container with the nuts into the container with the wet ingredients and blend together meticulously.

4. Make sure all dry ingredients get coated.

5. Put the granola mixture onto a parchment paper lined baking sheet and bake until the desired crunch is obtained roughly 8 to ten minutes.

6. Take off from the oven and allow to cool or eat hot.

7. Put ½ cup each Greek yogurt into two bowls.

8. Split the granola and drizzle over the yogurt in each container. Serve instantly.

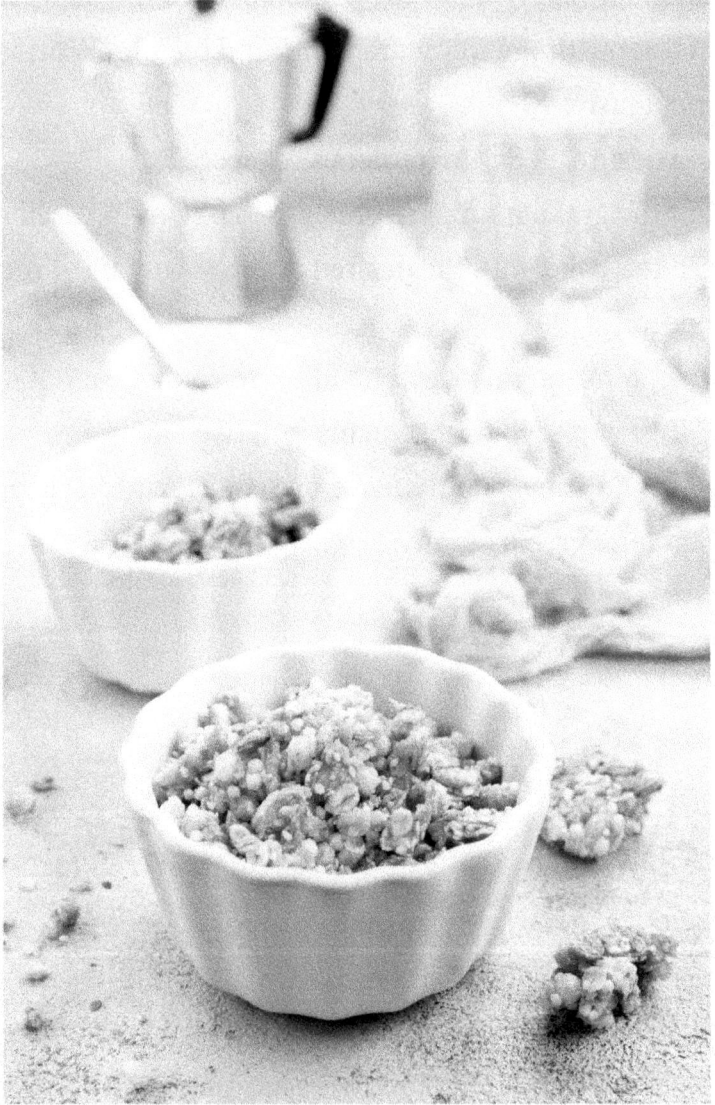

Coco-Tapioca Bowl

Time To Prepare: ten minutes

Time to Cook: twenty minutes

Yield: Servings 2

Ingredients:

- ¼ cup maple syrup
- ¼ cup tapioca pearls, small sized
- ½ cup unsweetened coconut flakes, toasted
- 1 ½ tsp. lemon juice
- 1 can light coconut milk
- 2 cups water

Directions:

1. Put the tapioca in a deep cooking pan and pour over the 2 cups of water.

2. Allow it to stand for a minimum 30 minutes.

3. Pour in the coconut milk and syrup and heat the deep cooking pan over moderate temperature.

4. Bring to its boiling point while stirring continuously.

5. Put in the lemon juice and stir and then decorate with coconut flakes.

Cranberry and Raisins Granola

Time To Prepare: fifteen minutes

Time to Cook: twenty minutes

Yield: Servings 4

Ingredients:
- 4 cups old-fashioned rolled oats
- 1 cup dried cranberries
- 1 cup golden raisins
- 2 tablespoons olive oil
- ½ cup almonds, slivered
- 2 tablespoons warm water
- 1 teaspoon vanilla extract
- 1 teaspoon cinnamon
- 6 tablespoons maple syrup
- 1/3 cup of honey
- 1/4 cup sesame seeds
- 1/4 teaspoon of salt
- 1/8 teaspoon nutmeg

Directions:
1. In a container, combine the sesame seeds, nutmeg, almonds, oats, salt, and cinnamon.

2. In another container, combine the oil, water, vanilla, honey, and syrup.

3. Slowly pour the mixture into the oats mixture. Toss to blend.

4. Spread the mixture into a greased jelly-roll pan.

5. Bake using your oven at 300°F for a minimum 55 minutes.

6. Stir and break the clumps every ten minutes.

7. Once you get it from the oven, stir the cranberries and raisins. Allow cooling.

8. This will last for a week when stored in an airtight container and up to a month when stored in your refrigerator.

Crepes with Coconut Cream & Strawberry Sauce

Time To Prepare: fifteen minutes

Time to Cook: 8 minutes

Yield: Servings 4

Ingredients:
For Sauce:

- 1 (13½-ounce) can chilled coconut milk
- 1 tablespoon honey
- 1 tablespoon organic honey
- 1 teaspoon organic vanilla flavoring
- 1½ teaspoons tapioca starch
- 12-ounces frozen strawberries, thawed and liquid reserved

For the Coconut cream: For Crepes:

- ¼ cup almond milk
- 2 organic eggs
- 2 tablespoons coconut flour
- 2 tablespoons tapioca starch Avocado oil, as required Pinch of salt

Directions:
For sauce inside a container,

1. Combine some reserved strawberry liquid and tapioca starch.

2. Put in the rest of the ingredients and mix thoroughly.

3. Move a combination inside a pan on moderate to high heat. Bring to its boiling point, stirring constantly.

4. Cook for minimum 2-3 minutes, till the sauce becomes thick.

5. Turn off the heat and aside, covered till serving.

For coconut cream,

1. Cautiously, scoop your cream from your surface of a can of coconut milk.

2. In a mixer, put in coconut cream, vanilla flavoring, and honey and pulse for around 6-8 minutes or till fluffy.

For crepes in a blender,

1. Put in all ingredients and pulse till well blended and smooth.

2. Lightly, grease a substantial non stick frying pan with avocado oil as well as heat on medium-low heat.

3. Put in a modest amount of mixture and tilt the pan to spread it uniformly inside the frying pan.

4. Cook roughly 1-2 minutes. Cautiously change the side and cook for roughly 1-1½ minutes more. Repeat with the rest of the mixture.

5. Split the coconut cream onto each crepe uniformly and fold into four equivalent portions.

6. Put strawberry sauce ahead before you serve.

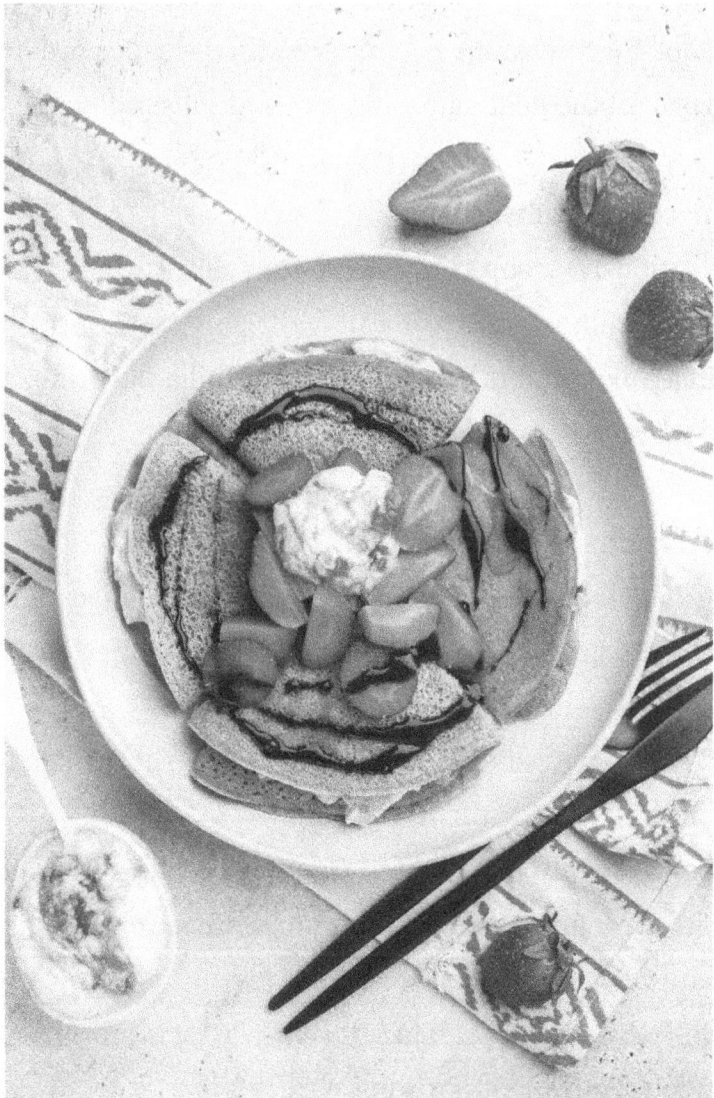

Egg Muffins with Feta and Quinoa

Time To Prepare: fifteen minutes

Time to Cook: thirty minutes

Yield: Servings 6-12

Ingredients:

- ¼ cup Black olives, chopped
- ¼ cup Onion, chopped
- ¼ tsp. Salt
- 1 cup Feta cheese
- 1 cup Quinoa, cooked
- 1 cup Tomatoes, chopped
- 1 tbsp. Oregano, fresh chop
- 2 cups baby spinach, chopped
- 2 tsp. Olive oil
- 8 Eggs

Directions:

1. Heat oven to 350.

2. Spray oil a muffin pan with twelve cups.

3. Cook spinach, oregano, olives, onion, and tomatoes for 5 minutes in the olive oil on moderate heat.

4. Beat eggs.

5. Put in the cooked mix of veggies to the eggs with the cheese and salt.

6. Ladle mix into muffin cups. Bake for thirty minutes.

These will remain fresh in your refrigerator for two days.

To eat, just wrap in a paper towel and warm in the microwave for thirty seconds.

Fennel Seeds Cookies

Time To Prepare: ten minutes

Time to Cook: twenty minutes

Yield: Servings 5

Ingredients:

- ¼ cup coconut oil, softened
- ¼ teaspoon whole fennel seeds
- ½ teaspoon fresh ginger, grated finely
- 1 teaspoon vanilla extract
- 1/3 cup coconut flour
- 2 tablespoons raw honey
- Pinch freshly ground black pepper
- Pinch of ground cinnamon
- Pinch of salt

Directions:

1. Set the oven to 360°F.

2. Coat a cookie sheet that has parchment paper.

3. In a substantial container, put in all together the ingredients and mix till a uniform dough form.

4. Form small balls in the mixture and put onto prepared cookie sheet inside a single layer.

5. Using your fingers, softly push along the balls to form the cookies.

6. Bake for minimum 9 minutes or till golden brown.

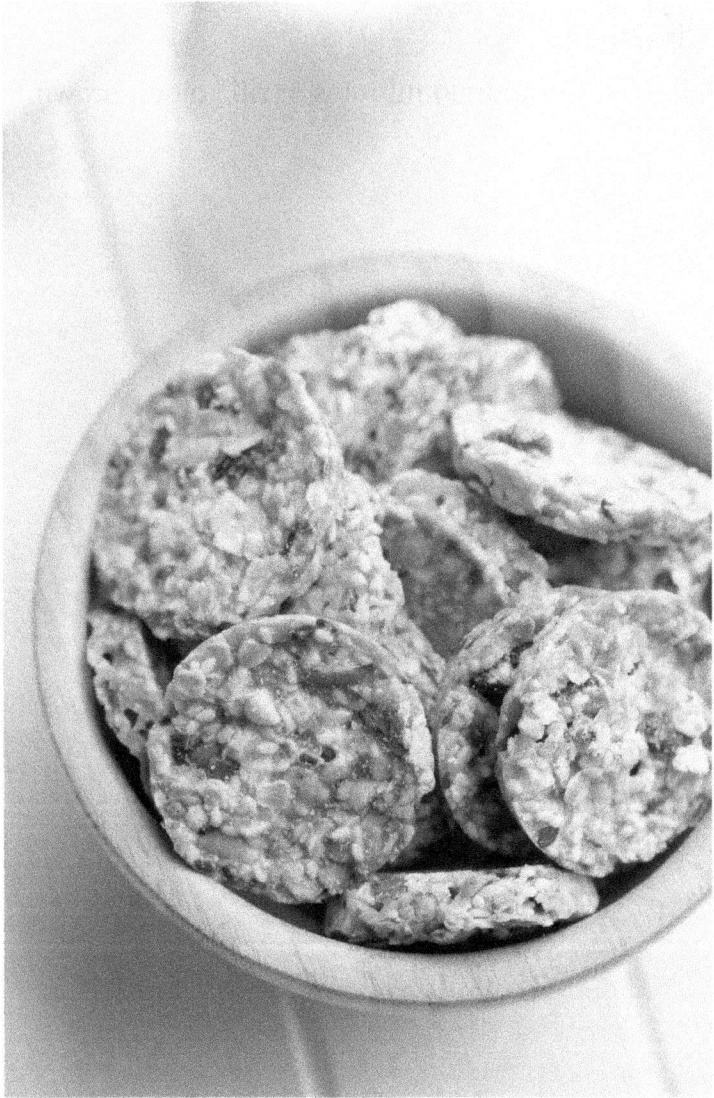

Fruity Muffins

Time To Prepare: ten minutes

Time to Cook: 2-3 minutes

Yield: Servings 8

Ingredients:

- ¼ cup brown rice flour
- ¼ cup extra-virgin olive oil
- ¼ cup raw sugar
- ½ cup almond meal
- ½ cup buckwheat flour
- ½ teaspoon ground ginger
- 1 big organic egg
- 1 cup rhubarb, cut finely
- 1 small apple, peeled, cored and chopped finely
- 1 tablespoon linseed meal
- 1 teaspoon organic vanilla extract
- 12 teaspoon ground cinnamon
- 2 tablespoons arrowroot flour
- 2 tablespoons crystallized ginger, chopped finely
- 2 tablespoons organic baking powder
- 7 tablespoons almond milk
- Pinch of salt

Directions:

1. Set the oven to 350F.

2. Grease 8 cups of a big muffin tin.

3. In a big container, combine almond meal, linseed meal, sugar, and crystalized ginger.

4. In another container, put together flours, baking powder, spices, and salt, and mix.

5. Sift the flour mixture into the container of almond meal mixture and mix thoroughly.

6. In a third container, put in egg, milk, oil, and vanilla and beat till well blended.

7. Put in egg mixture into the flour mixture and mix till well blended.

8. Fold in apple and rhubarb.

9. Put the mixture into prepared muffin cups equally.

10. Bake for approximately 20-twenty-five minutes or till a toothpick inserted in the middle comes out clean

Grapefruit-Pomegranate Salad

Time To Prepare: ten minutes

Time to Cook: 0 minutes

Yield: Servings 6

Ingredients:
- ¼ cup Basic Vegetable Stock
- 1 pomegranate
- 2 ruby red grapefruits
- 3 ounces Parmesan cheese
- 6 cups mesclun leaves

Directions:

1. Peel the grapefruit using a knife, take off all the pith. (the white layer under the skin).

2. Cut out every section with the knife, make sure that no pith remains.

3. Shave Parmesan using a vegetable peeler to make curls.

4. Peel the pomegranate using a paring knife; take off the berries/seeds.

5. Toss the mesclun greens in the stock.

6. To serve, mound the greens on plates and position the grapefruit sections, cheese, and pomegranate on top.

Ham and Veggie Frittata Muffins

Time To Prepare: ten minutes

Time to Cook: twenty-five minutes

Yield: Servings 12

Ingredients:

- ¼ cup coconut milk (canned)
- ½ yellow onion, finely diced
- 1 cup cherry tomatoes, halved
- 2 tablespoons coconut flour
- 4 tablespoons coconut oil
- 5 ounces thinly cut ham
- 8 big eggs
- 8 oz. frozen spinach, thawed and drained
- 8 oz. mushrooms, thinly cut
- Sea salt and pepper to taste

Directions:

1. Preheat your oven to 375 degrees Fahrenheit.

2. In a moderate-sized frying pan, warm the coconut oil on moderate heat.

3. Put in the onion and cook until tender.

4. Put in the mushrooms, spinach, and cherry tomatoes. Sprinkle with salt and pepper.

5. Cook until the mushrooms have become tender. About five minutes.

Turn off the heat and save for later.

6. In a huge container, beat the eggs with the coconut milk and coconut flour.

7. Mix in the cooled veggie mixture.

8. Coat each cavity of a 12 cavity muffin tin with the thinly cut ham.

9. Pour the egg mixture into each one and bake for about twenty minutes.

10. Take out of the oven and let cool for approximately five minutes before transferring to a wire rack.

Honey Pancakes

Time To Prepare: ten minutes

Time to Cook: five minutes

Yield: Servings 2

Ingredients:

- ¼ tsp baking soda
- ½ cup almond flour
- ½ tablespoon ground cinnamon
- ½ tablespoon ground ginger
- ½ tablespoon ground nutmeg
- ½ teaspoon ground cloves
- ½ teaspoon organic vanilla extract
- ¾ cup organic egg whites
- 1 tablespoon ground flaxseeds
- 2 tablespoons coconut flour
- 2 tablespoons organic honey
- Coconut oil, as required
- Pinch of salt

Directions:

1. In a big container, combine flours, flax seeds, baking soda, spices, and salt.

2. In another container, put in honey, egg whites and vanilla and beat till well blended.

3. Place the egg mixture into the flour mixture then mix till well blended.

4. Lightly, grease a big nonstick frying pan with oil and heat on medium-low heat.

5. Put in about ¼ cup of mixture and tilt the pan to spread it uniformly inside the frying pan.

6. Cook for approximately 3-4 minutes.

7. Cautiously, customize the side and cook roughly one minute more.

8. Repeat with the rest of the mixture.

9. Serve together with your desired topping.

Kale Turmeric Scramble

Time To Prepare: five minutes

Time to Cook: ten minutes

Yield: Servings 1

Ingredients:

- ¼ tsp. Black pepper
- ½ cup Kale, shredded
- ½ cup Sprouts
- 1 tbsp. Garlic, minced
- 1 tbsp. Turmeric, ground
- 2 Eggs
- 2 tbsp. Olive oil

Directions:

1. Beat the eggs and put in the turmeric, black pepper, and garlic.

2. Sauté the kale into the olive oil on moderate heat for 5 minutes, and then pour this egg mixture into the pan with the kale.

3. Carry on cooking, frequently stirring, until the eggs are cooked to your preference.

4. Top with raw sprouts before you serve.

Grams Mango Granola

Time To Prepare: ten minutes

Time to Cook: thirty minutes

Yield: Servings 4

Ingredients:

- ½ cup almonds, roughly chopped
- ½ cup dates, roughly chopped
- ½ cup nuts
- 1 cup dried mango, chopped
- 2 cups rolled oats
- 2 tbsp. coconut oil
- 2 tbsp. water
- 2 tsp. cinnamon
- 2/3 cup agave nectar
- 3 tbsp. sesame seeds

Directions:

1. Set oven at 320F In a big container, put the oats, almonds, nuts, sesame seeds, dates, and cinnamon then mix thoroughly.

2. In the meantime, heat a deep cooking pan on moderate heat, pour in the agave syrup, coconut oil, and water.

3. Stir and allow it to cook for minimum 3 minutes or until the coconut oil has melted.

4. Slowly pour the syrup mixture into the container with the oats and nuts and stir thoroughly, make sure that all the ingredients are coated with the syrup.

5. Move the granola on a baking sheet coated with parchment paper and place in your oven to bake for about twenty minutes.

6. After twenty minutes, take off the tray from the oven and lay the chopped dried mango on top.

7. Put back in your oven then bake again for another five minutes.

8. Allow the granola to cool completely before you serve or placing it in an airtight container for storage.

9. The shelf life of the granola will last up to 2-3 weeks.

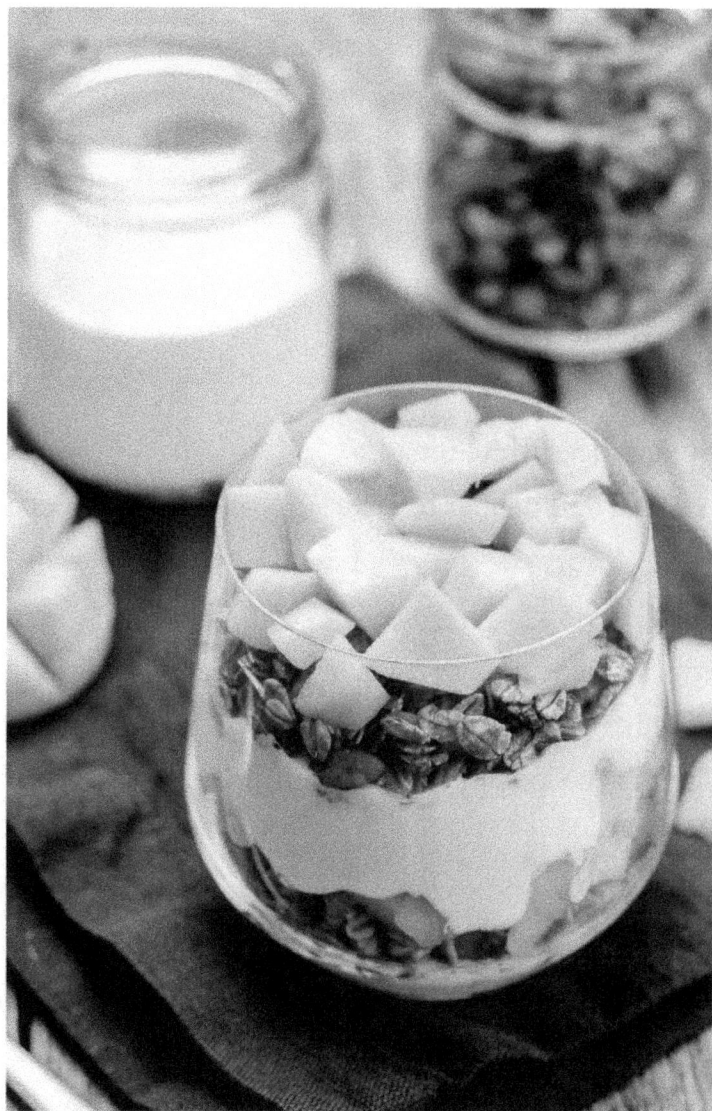

Maple Toast and Eggs

Time To Prepare: 20 Minutes

Time to Cook: 20 Minutes

Yield: Servings 6

Ingredients:
- ¼ cup butter
- ½ cup maple syrup
- 12 bacon strips, diced
- 12 big eggs
- 12 slices white bread
- Salt and pepper to taste

Directions:

1. Fry the bacon on a frying pan on moderate heat until the fat has rendered.

2. Take the bacon out and place it using paper towels to drain surplus fat.

3. Warm the maple syrup and butter until melted in a deep cooking pan. Set aside.

4. Trim the edges of the bread and flatten the slices with a rolling pin.

5. Brush one side with the syrup mixture and press the slices into greased muffin cups.

6. Split the bacon into the muffin cups.

7. Break one egg into each cup.

8. Drizzle with salt and pepper to taste

9. Cover using foil, then bake in your oven at 4000F for about twenty minutes or until the eggs have set

Mini Breakfast Pizza

Time To Prepare: 5 Minutes

Time to Cook: 10 Minutes

Yield: Servings 4

Ingredients:
- 4 eggs, beaten
- 2 English muffins, split and toasted
- ½ cup shredded Italian cheese
- Dried oregano leaves
- Cooking spray
- Salt and pepper to taste
- 1/3 cup commercial pizza sauce

Directions:
1. Preheat your oven to 4000F.

2. Coat a frying pan with cooking spray then heat on medium flame.

3. Flavour the eggs with salt and pepper to taste and pour into the frying pan.

4. As the eggs start to set, pull the eggs across the pan with an inverted turner.

5. Carry on cooking and folding the egg. Set aside.

6. Spread pizza sauce uniformly on English muffin halves and top with eggs and cheese.

7. Put on a baking sheet then bake for five minutes. Decorate using oregano last.

Nutty Oats Pudding

Time To Prepare: five minutes

Time to Cook: 0 minutes

Yield: Servings 3 -5

Ingredients:

- ¼ cup dry milk
- ¼ cup rolled oats
- ½ cup of water
- 1 ½ tablespoon natural peanut butter
- 1 tablespoon yogurt, fat-free
- 1 teaspoon peanuts, finely chopped

Directions:

1. Using a microwaveable-safe container, put together peanut butter and dry milk. Whisk well.

2. Put in water to achieve a smooth consistency. Put in oats.

3. Cover container using plastic wrap.

4. Create a small hole for the steam to escape.

5. Put inside the microwave oven for a minute on high powder.

6. Continue heating, this time on medium power for 90 seconds.

7. Allow to sit for five minutes.

8. To serve, spoon an equal amount of cereals in a container top with peanuts and yogurt.

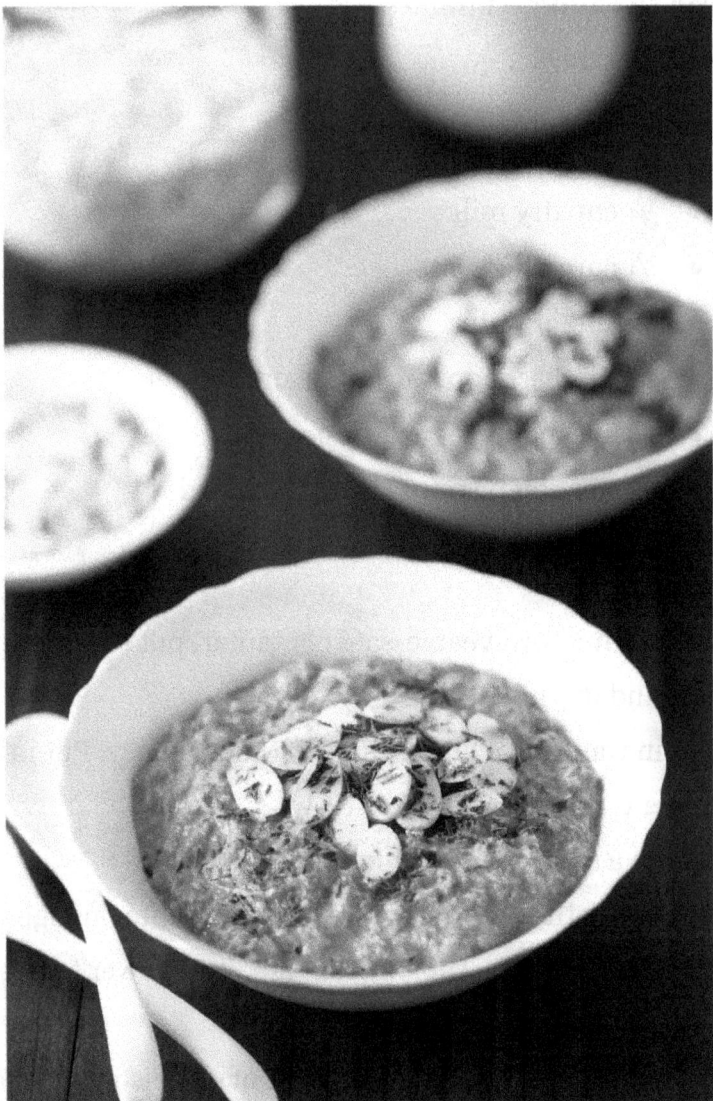

Oatmeal-Applesauce Muffins

Time To Prepare: fifteen minutes

Time to Cook: twenty-five minutes

Yield: Servings 12

Ingredients:

- Topping 1 tbsp. brown sugar
- 1 tbsp. unsalted butter, melted
- 1/4 cup rolled oats
- 1/8 tsp. cinnamon
- Muffins
- ½ c. brown sugar
- ½ c. unsweetened applesauce
- ½ tsp. Baking soda
- ½ tsp. Cinnamon
- ½ tsp. Salt
- ½ tsp. sugar
- 1 c. nonfat milk
- 1 c. old fashioned rolled oats (not instant)
- 1 c. whole wheat flour
- 1 tsp. Baking powder
- 2 egg whites raisins or nuts (opt.)

Directions:

1. To begin, first, pre soak the oats in milk for an hour, Set the oven to 400°F then grease a standard 12-cup muffin pan with cooking spray or use paper liners.

2. In a mixing container, mix oat-milk mixture, applesauce, and egg whites. Blend well and save for later.

3. In a different container, put together the whole wheat flour, brown sugar, baking powder, baking soda, salt, sugar, and cinnamon then mix.

4. Slowly put wet ingredients to dry ingredients and blend until just blended, but do not over mix the batter as it will make the muffins firm.

5. Put in raisins or nuts (opt.).

6. Prepare topping: In a small container, whisk together the oats, brown sugar, and cinnamon.

7. Put in melted butter and toss lightly using a fork to coat ingredients.

8. Fill each muffin cup 2/3 full of batter.

10. 9. Drizzle topping on the top of each batter-filled muffin cup.

11. Tap the pan gently on the counter to even out the batter.

12. Put muffin pan in preheated oven and cook for twenty to twenty-five minutes or until a toothpick put in the center of one of the muffins comes out clean.

13. Remove from the oven and allow it to sit for five minutes before you serve.

Banana Breakfast

Time To Prepare: ten minutes

Time to Cook: 0 minutes

Yield: Servings 2

Ingredients:

- ½ cup cold milk
- 1 big cut Banana
- 2 tbsp. flaxseeds
- 2 tbsp. ground coconut
- 4 tbsp. sesame seeds
- 4 tbsp. sunflower seeds

Directions:

1. Combine the milk and honey in your breakfast container.

2. Use your coffee grinder to grind all the seeds.

3. Put in the ground seeds to the honey and milk mixture.

4. Put the cut bananas neatly on top.

5. Drizzle the ground coconuts for added flavor.

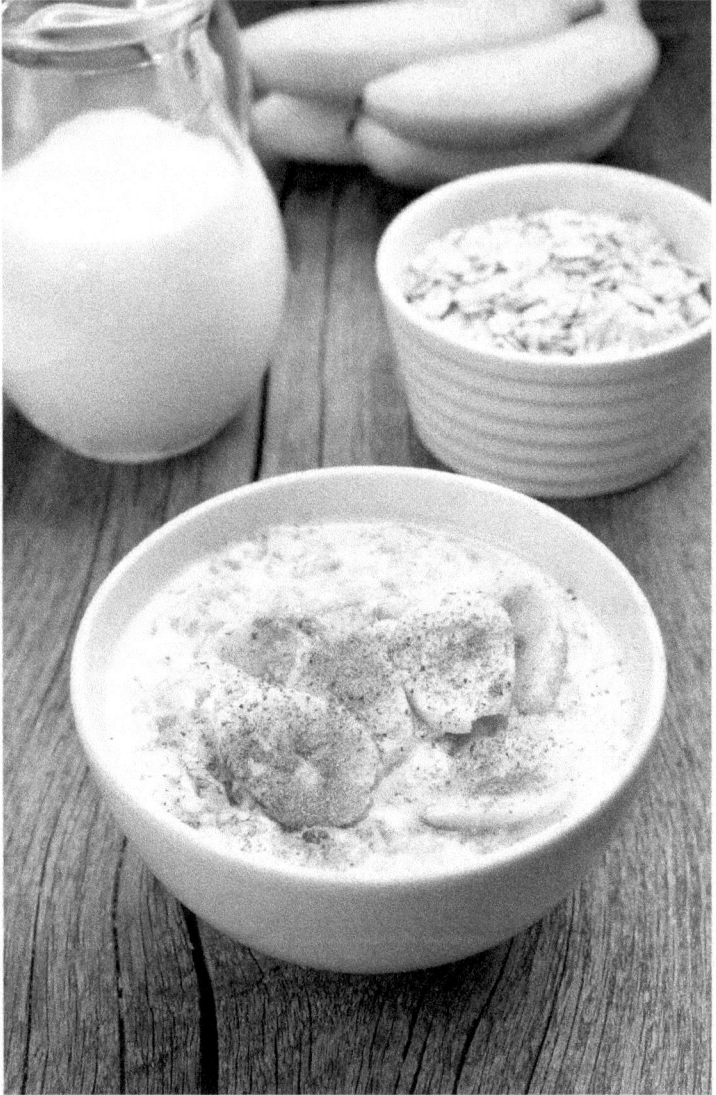

Peaches with Honey Almond Ricotta

Time To Prepare:fifteen minutes

Time to Cook: 0 minutes

Yield: Servings 4-6

Ingredients:

- ¼ cup Almond extract
- ¼ cup Peaches, cut
- ½ cup Almonds, thin slices
- 1 cup Ricotta, skim milk
- 1 tsp. Honey Bread, whole grain bagel or toast
- Spread To Serve

Directions:

1. Combine the almond extract, honey, ricotta, and almonds.

2. Spread one tablespoon of this mix on toasted bread and cover with peaches.

Poached Salmon Egg Toast

Time To Prepare: ten minutes

Time to Cook: 4 minutes

Yield: Servings 2

Ingredients:
- ¼ tsp. Black pepper
- ¼ tsp. Lemon juice
- 1 tbsp. Scallions, cut thin
- 1/8 tsp. Salt
- 2 Eggs, poached
- 2 tbs. Avocado, mashed
- 4 oz. Salmon, smoked Bread, two slices rye or whole-grain toasted

Directions:
1. Put in lemon juice to avocado with pepper and salt.

2. Spread the mixed avocado over the toasted bread slices.

3. Lay smoked salmon over toast and top with a poached egg. Top with cut scallions

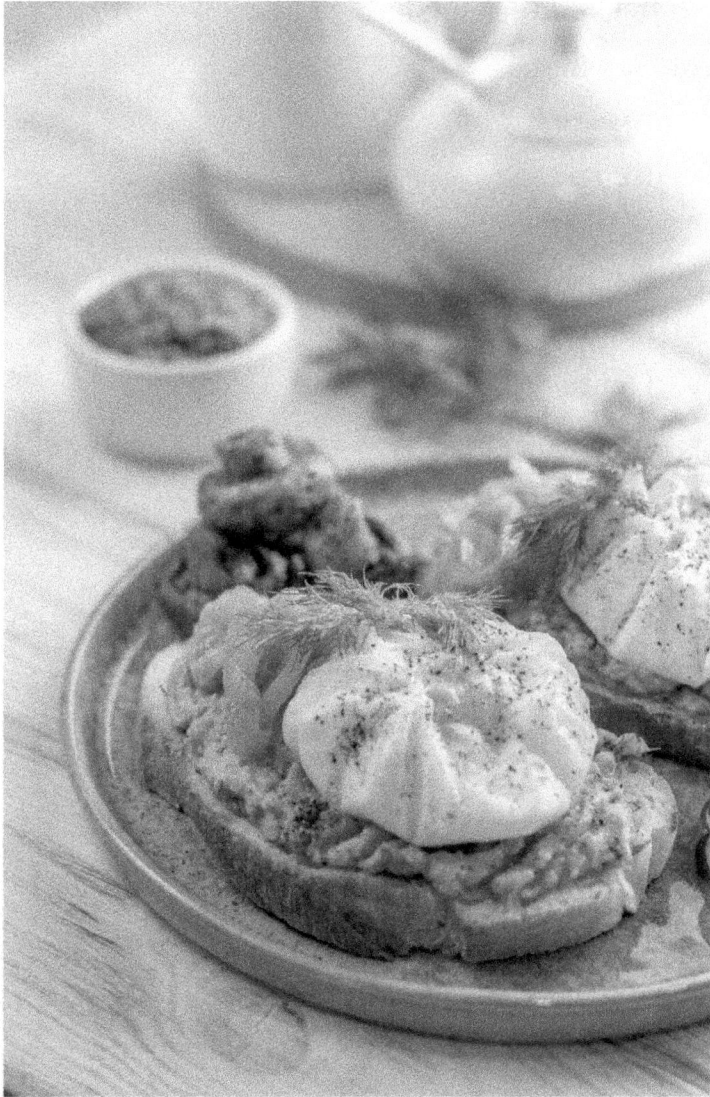

Pumpkin Pancakes

Time To Prepare: twenty-five minutes

Time to Cook: ten minutes

Yield: Servings 6

Ingredients:

- ½ cup pumpkin puree
- 1 cup coconut cream
- 1 ounce egg white Protein
- 1 tablespoon chai masala
- 1 tablespoon swerve
- 1 teaspoon baking powder
- 1 teaspoon coconut oil
- 1 teaspoon vanilla extract
- 2 ounces flax seeds; ground
- 2 ounces hazelnut flour
- 3 eggs
- 5 drops stevia

Directions:

1. In a container, mix flax seeds with hazelnut flour, egg white Protein baking powder and chai masala and stir.

2. In another container, mix coconut cream with vanilla extract, pumpkin puree, eggs, stevia, and swerve and stir thoroughly.

3. Mix the 2 mixtures and stir thoroughly.

4. Heat a pan with the oil on moderate to high heat; pour 1/6 of the batter, spread into a circle, cover, decrease the heat to low, cook for about three minutes on each side and move to a plate

5. Repeat the process using the rest of the mixture and serve pumpkin pancakes immediately.

Quinoa & Veggie Croquettes

Time To Prepare: fifteen minutes

Time to Cook: 9 minutes

Yield: Servings 12- fifteen

Ingredients:

- ¼ cup fresh cilantro leaves, chopped
- ¼ teaspoon ground turmeric
- ½ cup frozen peas, thawed
- 1 cup cooked quinoa
- 1 tbsp. essential olive oil
- 1 teaspoon garam masala
- 2 big boiled potatoes, peeled and mashed
- 2 minced garlic cloves
- 2 teaspoons ground cumin
- Freshly ground black pepper, to taste
- Olive oil, for frying Salt, to taste

Directions:

1. In a frying pan, warm oil on moderate heat.

2. Put in peas and garlic and sauté for approximately one minute.

3. Move the pea mixture into a big container.

4. Put in the remaining ingredients and mix till well blended.

5. Make equal sized oblong shaped patties from your mixture.

6. In a huge frying pan, heat oil on moderate to high heat.

7. Put in croquettes and fry for approximately 4 minutes per side.

Quinoa Breakfast Bowl

Time To Prepare: thirty minutes

Time to Cook: 0 minutes

Yield: Servings 6

Ingredients:

- ¼ cup Greek yogurt, plain
- ½ tsp. Salt
- 1 cup Baby spinach, chopped
- 1 cup Feta cheese
- 1 Pint Cherry tomatoes, cut in halves
- 1 tsp. Black pepper
- 1 tsp. Garlic, minced
- 1 tsp. Olive oil
- 12 Eggs
- 2 cups Quinoa, cooked

Directions:

1. Mix together the eggs, salt, pepper, garlic, onion powder, and yogurt.

2. Cook the spinach and tomatoes for 5 minutes in the olive oil on moderate heat.

3. Pour in the egg mix and stir until eggs have set to your preferred doneness.

4. Stir in quinoa and feta until they are hot.

5. This will store in your refrigerator for two to three days.

Salmon Burgers

Time To Prepare: fifteen minutes

Time to Cook: 8 minutes

Yield: Servings 3

Ingredients:
- ½ of a medium onion, chopped
- 1 (6-oz. can) skinless, boneless salmon, drained
- 1 celery rib, chopped
- 1 tablespoon dried dill, crushed
- 1 tablespoon plus 1 teaspoon coconut flour
- 1 teaspoon lemon
- 2 big eggs
- 3 tablespoons coconut oil
- Freshly ground black pepper, to taste
- Salt, to taste

Directions:

1. In a substantial container, put in salmon and which has a fork, break it into little pieces.

2. Put in rest of the ingredients excluding the for oil and mix till well blended.

3. Make 6 equal sized small patties from the mixture.

4. In a substantial frying pan, melt coconut oil on moderate to high heat.

5. Cook the patties for about four minutes per side.

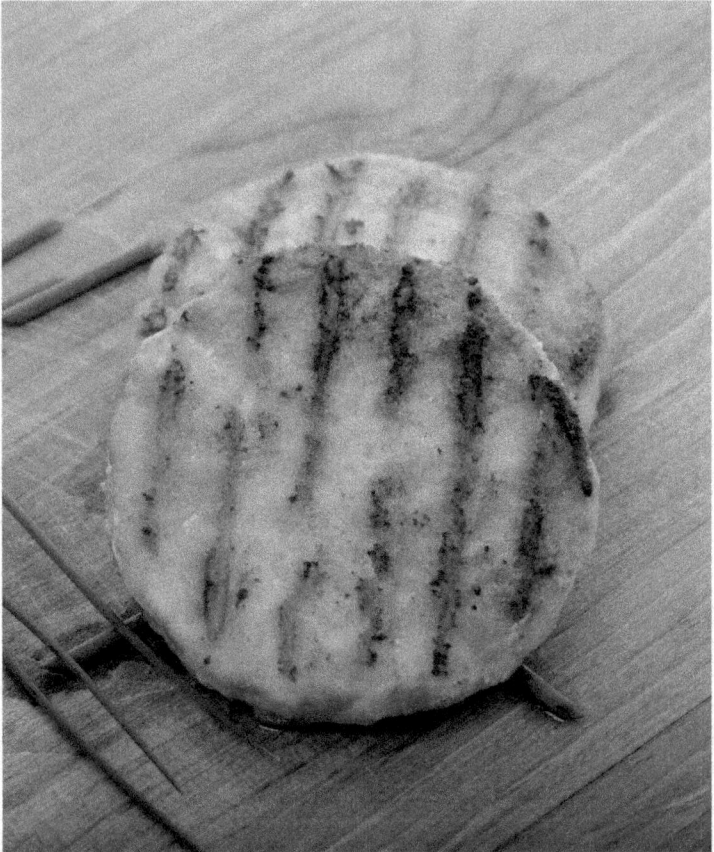

Savory Bread

Time To Prepare: ten minutes

Time to Cook: 20 minutes

Yield: Servings 8-10

Ingredients:

- ½ cup plus 1tablespoon almond flour
- 1 cup raw cashew butter
- 1 tablespoon apple cider vinegar
- 1 tablespoon water
- 1 teaspoon ground turmeric
- 1 tsp. baking soda
- 2 big organic eggs
- 2 organic egg whites
- Salt, to taste

Directions:

1. Set the oven to 350F. Grease a loaf pan.

2. In a big pan, combine flour, baking soda, turmeric, and salt. In another container, put in eggs, egg whites, and cashew butter and beat till smooth.

3. Slowly, put in water and beat till well blended.

4. Put in flour mixture and mix till well blended.

5. Mix in apple cider vinegar treatment.

6. Put the combination into prepared loaf pan uniformly.

7. Bake for around 20 minutes or till a toothpick inserted within the middle is released clean.

Shirataki Pasta with Avocado and Cream

Time To Prepare: ten minutes

Time to Cook: six minutes

Yield: Servings 2

Ingredients:

- ½ of an avocado
- ½ packet of shirataki noodles, cooked
- ½ tsp cracked black pepper
- ½ tsp dried basil
- ½ tsp salt
- 1/8 cup heavy cream

Directions:

1. Put a medium pot half full with water on moderate heat, bring it to boil, then put in noodles and cook for a couple of minutes.

2. Then drain the noodles and set aside until required.

3. Put avocado in a container, purée it using a fork, Mash avocado in a container, move it to a blender, put in rest of the ingredients, and pulse until the desired smoothness is achieved.

4. Take a frying pan, place it on moderate heat and when hot, put in noodles in it, pour in the avocado mixture, stir thoroughly and cook for a couple of minutes until hot.

5. Serve straight away.

Spicy Marble Eggs

Time To Prepare: fifteen minutes

Time to Cook: 2 hours

Yield: Servings 12

Ingredients:

- 1 dried cinnamon stick, whole
- 1 thumb-sized fresh ginger, unpeeled, crushed
- 1 tsp. dried Szechuan peppercorns
- 1 tsp. salt
- 2 dried bay leaves
- 2 oolong black tea bags
- 3 dried star anise, whole
- 3 Tbsp. brown sugar
- 3 Tbsp. light soy sauce
- 4 cups of water
- 4 Tbsp. dark soy sauce
- 6 medium-boiled eggs, unpeeled, cooled For the Marinade

Directions:

1. Use the back of a spoon to crack eggshells in places to create a spider web effect. Do not peel. Set aside until needed.

2. Pour marinade into a big Dutch oven set using high heat. Put the lid partly on.

3. Bring water to a rolling boil, approximately five minutes. Turn off heat. Close the lid.

4. Steep ingredients for about ten minutes. Use a slotted spoon to fish out and discard solids.

5. Cool marinade completely to room proceeding.

6. Put eggs into an airtight non-reactive container just small enough to tightly fit all these in. 7. Pour in marinade. Eggs must be completely immersed in liquid. Discard leftover marinade, if any.

8. Coat container rim with generous layers of saran wrap. Secure container lid.

9. Chill eggs for one day before you use them.

10. Extract eggs and drain each piece well before you use, but keep the rest immersed in the marinade.

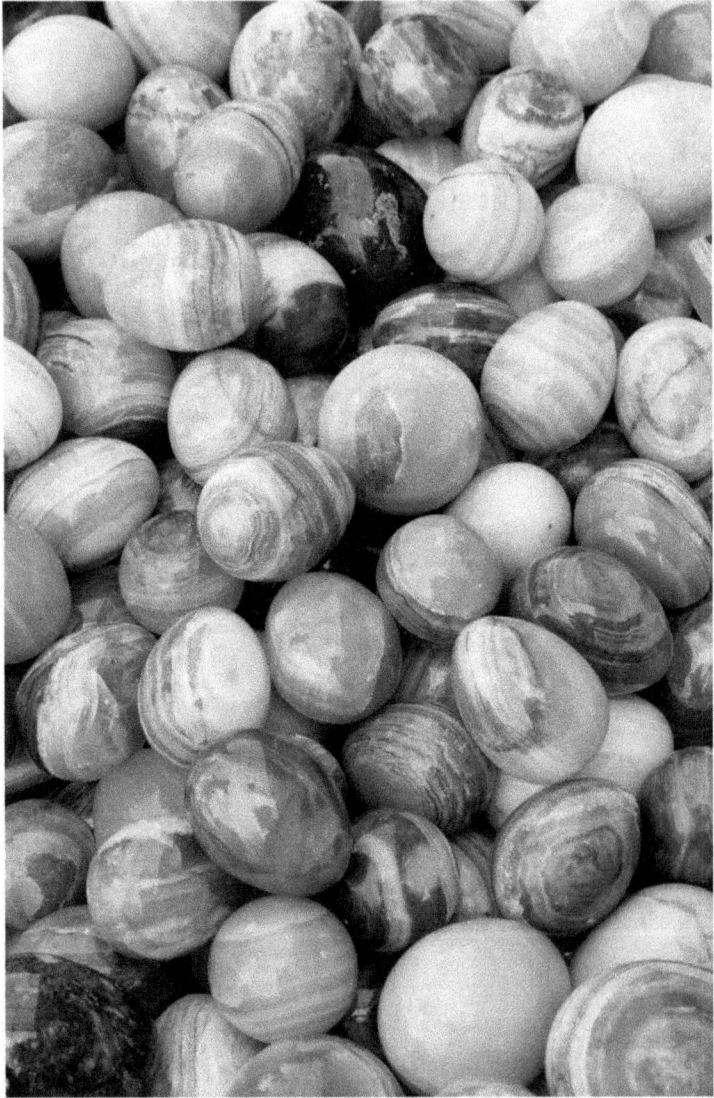

Spinach Mushroom Omelet

Time To Prepare: three minutes

Time to Cook: fifteen minutes

Yield: Servings 2

Ingredients:

- ¼ cup Red onion, diced
- ½ Spinach, fresh, chopped
- ½ tsp. Salt
- 1 Green onion, diced
- 1 oz. Feta cheese
- 1 tbsp. Olive oil
- 3 Egg
- 5 Mushrooms, button, cut

Directions:

1. Sauté the mushrooms, onions, and spinach for four minutes and set them aside.

2. Beat eggs meticulously and pour into the frying pan.

3. Cook for three to four minutes until edges start to turn brown.

4. Drizzle all other ingredients onto half of the omelet and fold the other half over.

5. Cook the omelet for a minute on each side.

Strawberry Yogurt treat

Time To Prepare: ten minutes

Time to Cook: 0 minutes

Yield: Servings 2

Ingredients:

- 1 cup cut strawberries
- 4 cups 0% Fat plain yogurt
- 4 tbsp. honey
- 8 tbsp. of flax meal
- 8 tbsp. walnuts (chopped)

Directions:

1. Distribute 2 cups of the yogurt into your serving bowls.

2. Neatly layer the flax meal and the walnut in the center.

3. Put in a sprinkle of half of the honey before covering with the final layer of yogurt.

4. Put in the honey on top of the yogurt to put in color when you serve.

Sun-Dried Tomato Garlic Bruschetta

Time To Prepare: ten minutes

Time to Cook: five minutes

Yield: Servings 6

Ingredients:
- 1 garlic clove, peeled
- 1 tsp. chives, minced
- 1 tsp. olive oil
- 2 slices sourdough bread, toasted
- 2 tsp. sun-dried tomatoes in olive oil, minced

Directions:

1. Vigorously rub garlic clove on 1 side of each of the toasted bread slices

2. Spread equivalent portions of sun-dried tomatoes on the garlic side of bread.

3. Drizzle chives and sprinkle olive oil on top.

4. Pop both slices into oven toaster, and cook until well thoroughly heated.

5. Put bruschetta on a plate.

6. Serve warm

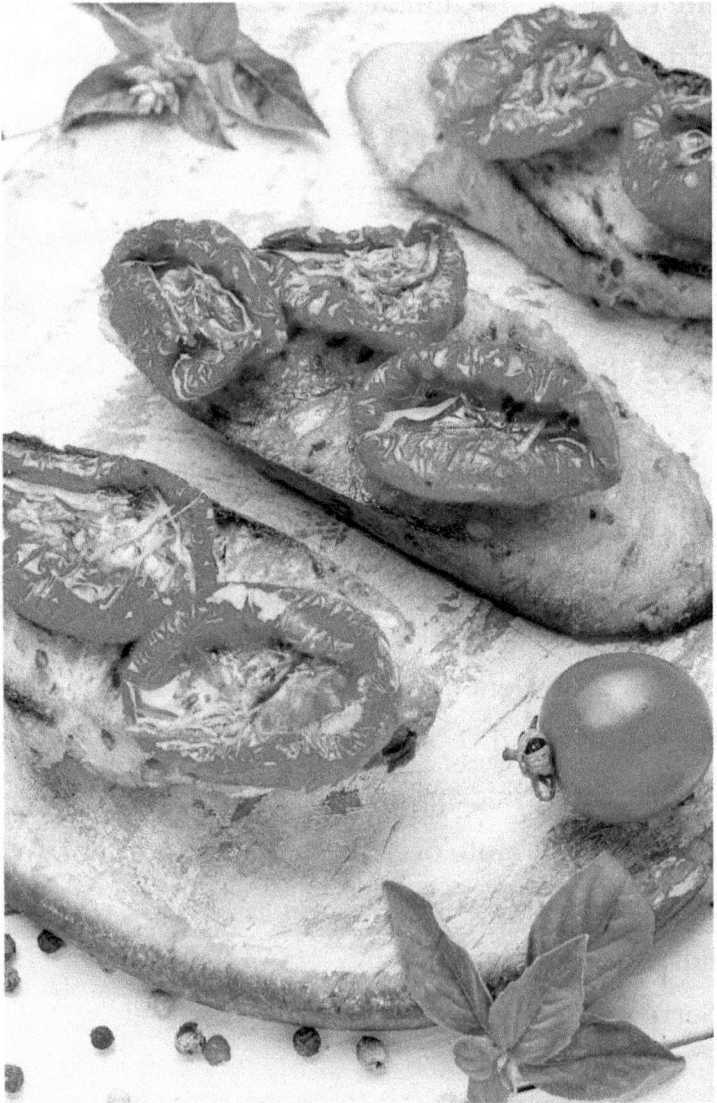

Notes

www.ingramcontent.com/pod-product-compliance
Lightning Source LLC
Chambersburg PA
CBHW050800030426
42336CB00012B/1880